Mindfulness Meditation for Brain Cancer Patients

Finding Inner Peace Amidst the Storm

Copyright Notice

Disclaimer

This book falls within the realm of nonfiction in the field of health. The information presented here is intended solely for general informational purposes and should not be considered a replacement for professional medical advice, diagnosis, or treatment. It is imperative to always seek guidance from a qualified healthcare provider or physician regarding any inquiries you may have about a medical condition. Please do not disregard professional medical advice or delay seeking it based on the content found in this book.

Contents

Introduction

In the face of adversity, the human spirit possesses a remarkable capacity for resilience and renewal. When confronted with the harrowing diagnosis of brain cancer, individuals and their loved ones often find themselves caught in a tempest of fear, uncertainty, and emotional turbulence. This is a storm that, for all its chaos, can reveal profound inner strength and wisdom. It is within the darkest moments that the light of mindfulness meditation can shine most brilliantly.

In "Mindfulness Meditation for Brain Cancer Patients: Finding Inner Peace Amidst the Storm," we embark on a journey of healing, hope, and self-discovery. This book is a testament to the human spirit's unwavering potential to find tranquility amidst the most tumultuous circumstances. Brain cancer is a formidable foe, but with the powerful tool of mindfulness, we can find a sanctuary of calm within the tempest.

In these pages, we will explore the profound ways in which mindfulness meditation can offer solace, strength, and clarity to those facing brain cancer. We will delve into the science behind mindfulness and its remarkable benefits for managing the physical and emotional challenges that cancer presents. More importantly, we will guide you through practical techniques and exercises that can be integrated into daily life, helping you nurture your inner peace and resilience.

This book is a beacon of hope. It is an invitation to embark on a journey of self-compassion and self-discovery. As we navigate the labyrinth of brain cancer, mindfulness becomes the guiding light that illuminates our path, offering a sense of control and serenity even when the world around us feels uncontrollable.

Whether you are a patient, caregiver, friend, or family member, this book is a source of support for anyone whose life has been touched by brain cancer. Our aim is not to negate the storm but to show you how to find peace within it, how to become the eye of the hurricane and, in that stillness, discover the strength and resilience you never knew you possessed.

Together, we will explore the transformative power of mindfulness meditation as we embark on this journey toward finding inner peace amidst the storm.

Chapter 1

Understanding Brain Cancer

The human brain is a marvel of complexity and function, yet it is also susceptible to diseases that can be devastating. Brain cancer, one such affliction, poses a unique challenge due to the critical role the brain plays in our daily lives. In this chapter, we will delve into the world of brain cancer, exploring the types of brain cancer, the methods of diagnosis and staging, and the conventional treatments available along with their associated side effects.

Types of Brain Cancer

Brain cancer, also known as brain tumor, refers to the abnormal and uncontrollable growth of cells within the brain. These tumors can be broadly classified into two main categories: primary brain tumors and metastatic brain tumors.

1. **Primary Brain Tumors**: These tumors originate in the brain itself and are the more common type of brain cancer. They can be further categorized into benign and malignant tumors. Benign tumors are non-cancerous and tend to grow slowly, often causing symptoms due to their size and pressure on surrounding brain tissue. Malignant tumors are cancerous and grow more aggressively.

a. **Gliomas**: Gliomas are a subset of primary brain tumors that originate from glial cells, which are the supporting cells of the central nervous system. These tumors can be both benign (non-cancerous) and malignant (cancerous) and are the most common primary brain tumors in adults. Understanding gliomas is essential as they encompass a wide range of tumor types with varying characteristics and treatment approaches.

Types of Gliomas:

Gliomas are categorized into several subtypes, each with distinct characteristics:

- **Astrocytomas:** These gliomas arise from astrocytes, a type of glial cell. They can be slow-growing (low-grade) or more aggressive (high-grade). Glioblastoma multiforme, a high-grade astrocytoma, is one of the most aggressive and common forms of primary brain cancer.

- **Oligodendrogliomas:** Oligodendrogliomas develop from oligodendrocytes, another type of glial cell. They tend to be slow-growing and are often found in the frontal lobes of the brain.

- **Ependymomas:** These gliomas originate from ependymal cells lining the brain's ventricles and central canal. They are more common in children and young adults.

- **Mixed Gliomas**: These tumors contain a mixture of cell types, such as both astrocytic and oligodendroglial components.

b. **Meningiomas**: Meningiomas are a type of primary brain tumor that develops in the meninges, which are the protective membranes surrounding the brain and spinal cord. These tumors are typically slow-growing and are usually benign (non-cancerous). Meningiomas are the most common type of brain tumor in adults, and understanding them is crucial as they have distinct characteristics and require appropriate management.

Characteristics of Meningiomas:

- **Benign Nature:** The majority of meningiomas are benign and do not invade the brain tissue. They grow on the surface of the brain, often pushing against it.

- **Slow Growth:** Meningiomas tend to grow slowly over time. Some may remain small and asymptomatic for years, while others can become larger and cause symptoms.

- **Location:** Meningiomas can arise in various areas of the brain and spinal cord, depending on where the meninges are located. The most common locations include the convexity of the brain, parasagittal region, olfactory groove, and the base of the skull.

2. **Metastatic Brain Tumors:**

Metastatic brain tumors, also known as secondary brain tumors or brain metastases, are cancerous growths that develop in the brain as a result of cancer cells that have spread (metastasized) from another primary cancer site in the body. These tumors are different from primary brain tumors, which originate in the brain itself. Metastatic brain tumors are a significant concern in cancer care and require specialized treatment and management.

Characteristics of Metastatic Brain Tumors:

- **Origins**: Metastatic brain tumors result from the migration of cancer cells from a primary cancer site elsewhere in the body. Common primary cancer sites that can lead to brain metastases include the lungs, breast, kidney, colon, and skin (melanoma).

- **Number and Location**: Metastatic brain tumors can be solitary or multiple and can occur in various regions of the brain. They are named based on their primary cancer site, such as lung metastases or breast metastases.

Diagnosis and Staging

Diagnosis and staging of brain cancer are critical processes in determining the type, location, extent, and severity of brain tumors. Accurate diagnosis and staging help guide treatment decisions and provide crucial information for prognosis. Here's an overview of how brain cancer is diagnosed and staged:

1. Clinical Evaluation:

- **Medical History**: The process begins with a detailed medical history, where the patient's symptoms, family medical history, and any relevant risk factors are discussed.

- **Physical Examination**: A neurological examination is conducted to assess the patient's motor and sensory functions, coordination, reflexes, and cognitive abilities.

2. Imaging Studies:

- **MRI (Magnetic Resonance Imaging)**: MRI is the primary imaging technique used to visualize brain tumors. It provides detailed images of the brain's structures and helps identify the tumor's size, location, and characteristics.

- **CT (Computed Tomography) Scan**: CT scans may also be used to provide additional information, particularly in emergencies when an MRI is not immediately available.

3. Biopsy:

- **Surgical Biopsy**: A sample of the tumor is obtained through surgery, allowing for the examination of tumor cells under a microscope. This helps determine the tumor type and grade.

- **Needle Biopsy**: In some cases, a less invasive needle biopsy may be used to obtain a tissue sample for analysis.

4. Laboratory Tests:

- **Molecular and Genetic Testing**: Molecular and genetic analysis of the tumor tissue can reveal specific mutations and markers, which can guide treatment decisions.

5. Staging:

Brain tumors are not typically staged like other cancers, using the TNM system. Instead, they are classified based on grade and extent:

- **Grade**: Brain tumors are categorized by grade, which reflects their aggressiveness. The World Health Organization (WHO) grades brain tumors from I to IV, with Grade I being the least aggressive (typically benign) and Grade IV being the most aggressive (highly malignant).

- **Extent of Spread**: The extent of tumor spread within the brain is typically described as localized (confined to a specific area) or diffuse (spread throughout the brain).

6. Additional Diagnostic Procedures:

- **Cerebrospinal Fluid Analysis:** In some cases, a lumbar puncture (spinal tap) is performed to analyze cerebrospinal fluid for signs of cancer cells or other abnormalities.

- **Functional Imaging:** Functional MRI (fMRI) and positron emission tomography (PET) scans can help identify regions of the brain involved in critical functions like speech and movement.

7. Staging of Metastatic Brain Tumors:

If the brain tumor is a metastatic tumor originating from another site in the body, the primary cancer's stage is considered when making treatment decisions.

8. Multidisciplinary Review:

Diagnosis and staging are typically done in collaboration with a team of medical professionals, including neurosurgeons, oncologists, radiologists, and pathologists, to ensure a comprehensive evaluation and to determine the most suitable treatment plan.

Accurate diagnosis and staging are crucial for selecting the most appropriate treatment, whether it's surgery, radiation therapy, chemotherapy, targeted therapy, or a combination of these modalities. Treatment decisions are also influenced by the patient's overall health and the specific characteristics of the brain tumor.

Conventional Treatments and Their Side Effects

Conventional treatments for brain cancer can vary depending on the type of brain tumor, its location, size, and grade. The main treatment modalities include surgery, radiation therapy, and chemotherapy. While these treatments are effective in controlling and managing brain cancer, they can also be associated with various side effects. Here's an overview of each treatment and their potential side effects:

1. Surgery:

Treatment: Surgical resection aims to remove as much of the brain tumor as safely possible. In some cases, complete removal is not achievable due to the tumor's location.

Side Effects:

- **Neurological Deficits**: Depending on the tumor's location, patients may experience post-operative neurological deficits, such as weakness, speech problems, or memory issues.

- **Infection**: Surgical procedures carry a risk of infection, which can be localized or systemic.

- **Hemorrhage**: There is a risk of bleeding during surgery, which can lead to complications.

- **Swelling**: Brain tissue can swell after surgery, leading to increased intracranial pressure.

2. Radiation Therapy:

Treatment: Radiation therapy, which includes external beam radiation and stereotactic radiosurgery, targets and destroys cancer cells in the brain.

Side Effects:

- **Fatigue**: Patients often experience fatigue, which can be persistent during and after treatment.

- **Hair Loss**: Hair loss is possible, but it's typically limited to the area receiving radiation.

- **Skin Changes**: The skin in the radiation area can become red, dry, or irritated.

- **Cognitive Changes**: Some patients may experience memory and cognitive changes, particularly with whole-brain radiation.

- **Swelling**: Brain tissue can swell in response to radiation, causing symptoms.

3. Chemotherapy:

Treatment: Chemotherapy involves the use of drugs that target and kill cancer cells, often administered systemically through the bloodstream.

Side Effects:

- **Nausea and Vomiting**: Chemotherapy is notorious for causing nausea and vomiting, which can be managed with anti-nausea medications.

- **Fatigue**: Patients often experience fatigue during chemotherapy.

- **Low Blood Counts**: Chemotherapy can reduce the number of white blood cells, red blood cells, and platelets, increasing the risk of infection, anemia, and bleeding.

- **Hair Loss**: Some chemotherapy drugs can lead to hair loss.

- **Neuropathy**: Peripheral neuropathy can cause numbness and tingling in the hands and feet.

- **Cognitive Changes**: Sometimes referred to as "chemo brain," chemotherapy can lead to memory and cognitive issues.

- **Mouth and Gastrointestinal Issues**: Sore mouth, mouth ulcers, and gastrointestinal problems are common side effects.

It's important to note that the specific side effects and their severity can vary depending on the individual, the type of treatment, and the combination of treatments used. Moreover, advances in medical management and supportive care have led to better management and reduction of side effects associated with these conventional treatments. Patients should work closely with their medical team to manage and mitigate any potential side effects during their brain cancer treatment.

Chapter 2

Mind-Body Connection: How Mindfulness Affects Healing

The mind-body connection is a powerful and complex phenomenon, which has gained substantial recognition in the realm of cancer care. Among the various practices and approaches that have emerged, mindfulness stands out as a valuable tool that can profoundly impact the journey of those facing cancer. In this chapter, we will explore the profound relationship between mindfulness and healing, with a specific focus on its relevance to cancer patients.

The Essence of Mindfulness

The essence of mindfulness is a profound and ancient concept that has gained significant attention in recent years, particularly in the fields of psychology, wellness, and self-improvement. At its core, mindfulness is a state of being fully present in the moment, observing and experiencing each moment without judgment or distraction. It is a mental practice and a way of life that can have a transformative impact on our overall well-being.

Key aspects of the essence of mindfulness include:

1. **Present-Moment Awareness:** Mindfulness involves focusing your attention on the present moment, which

means letting go of worries about the past or anxieties about the future. This awareness can be applied to all aspects of life, from mundane tasks to profound experiences.

2. **Non-Judgmental Acceptance:** In mindfulness, there is no judgment of whether a thought or emotion is "good" or "bad." It encourages a non-reactive, non-judgmental attitude towards your thoughts, feelings, and sensations. This acceptance can lead to a more balanced and compassionate perspective.

3. **Attention and Concentration:** Mindfulness requires conscious effort to direct your attention to the object of focus, whether it's your breath, bodily

sensations, or the sights and sounds around you. It cultivates a heightened level of concentration.

4. **Emotional Regulation:** Through mindfulness, individuals learn to observe their emotions and thoughts without immediate reaction. This can lead to better emotional regulation and a reduction in impulsive behavior.

5. **Stress Reduction**: One of the most widely recognized benefits of mindfulness is its ability to reduce stress. By staying in the present moment and letting go of worries, individuals can experience a greater sense of calm and relaxation.

6. **Improved Mental Health:** Mindfulness practices have been shown to be

beneficial for individuals dealing with anxiety, depression, and other mental health challenges. It can help in managing symptoms and promoting mental resilience.

7. **Enhanced Physical Well-Being:** Mindfulness has been linked to various physical health benefits, such as lower blood pressure, improved sleep, and enhanced immune function. It can also promote a healthier lifestyle by encouraging mindful eating and exercise.

8. **Interpersonal Relationships:** Mindfulness can improve the quality of relationships by fostering better communication, empathy, and active listening.

9. **Spiritual Growth**: For some, mindfulness is a spiritual practice that helps connect them to a deeper sense of self and the world around them.

The essence of mindfulness can be cultivated through various techniques, including meditation, deep breathing exercises, and mindful walking. Mindfulness can be incorporated into daily life, from being mindful while eating to practicing mindfulness in workplace settings.

Ultimately, the essence of mindfulness lies in the ability to engage with the present moment with full awareness, acceptance, and compassion. It is a powerful tool for personal growth, self-discovery, and well-being, helping individuals live more fulfilling lives by savoring each moment and finding peace in the midst of life's challenges.

The Cancer-Mindfulness Connection

The cancer-mindfulness connection refers to the practice of mindfulness and its potential benefits for cancer patients, both in terms of managing the physical and emotional challenges of cancer and enhancing the overall quality of life. This connection has gained attention in the field of oncology and complementary medicine. Here are some key aspects of the cancer-mindfulness connection:

1. Stress Reduction: A cancer diagnosis and its subsequent treatments can be incredibly stressful. Mindfulness techniques, including meditation and deep breathing, have been shown to reduce stress and anxiety levels. By practicing mindfulness, cancer patients can learn to manage their emotional responses to the disease, potentially improving their mental well-being.

2. **Pain Management**: Mindfulness has been found to be effective in reducing the perception of pain and improving pain management for cancer patients. By focusing on the present moment and observing sensations without judgment, individuals can develop a greater sense of control over their pain experience.

3. **Improved Emotional Well-Being**: Cancer can lead to a range of emotions, from fear and sadness to anger and frustration.

Mindfulness can help individuals acknowledge and cope with these emotions without becoming overwhelmed. It encourages self-compassion and emotional resilience.

4. Enhanced Quality of Life: The cancer-mindfulness connection can contribute to an overall improvement in the quality of life for cancer patients. It promotes a greater sense of well-being, helping individuals find moments of joy and meaning even during challenging times.

5. Better Sleep: Many cancer patients experience sleep disturbances, which can exacerbate other symptoms and diminish their quality of life. Mindfulness techniques can improve sleep quality by reducing nighttime rumination and anxiety.

6. Coping with Uncertainty: A cancer diagnosis often comes with uncertainty and fear of the future. Mindfulness can teach individuals to accept uncertainty and focus on what is within their control. This can lead to a more adaptive and less anxious approach to the challenges of cancer.

7. Encouraging Mindful Self-Care: Mindfulness practices promote self-care and self-compassion. Cancer patients can learn to prioritize their own well-being and take better care of themselves throughout the treatment process.

8. Supportive Community: Engaging in mindfulness practices, such as group meditation sessions, can foster a sense of community and support among cancer patients and survivors. This connection can be an essential aspect of emotional healing.

9. **Complementary to Conventional Treatments:** The cancer-mindfulness connection is not a replacement for conventional cancer treatments but can be a valuable complement. Many cancer centers and healthcare providers offer mindfulness-based programs as part of comprehensive cancer care.

10. **Positive Impact on Physical Health:** There is evidence that mindfulness practices may have a positive impact on physical health, such as reducing inflammation and enhancing the immune system. This can support the body's ability to cope with

cancer and treatment-related side effects. While mindfulness can offer many benefits to cancer patients, it's important to note that its effectiveness may vary from person to person. It's advisable for cancer patients to consult with healthcare professionals and seek guidance from experienced mindfulness practitioners to determine the most appropriate practices and techniques for their specific needs and circumstances.

The mind-body connection and the role of mindfulness in healing are profound, especially in the context of cancer. This practice empowers individuals facing cancer to better navigate the emotional, physical, and psychological challenges that accompany a diagnosis. By embracing mindfulness as part of their journey, cancer patients can not only enhance their quality of life but also strengthen their capacity for resilience and healing, ultimately leading to a more holistic and balanced approach to cancer care.

Chapter 3

Starting Your Mindfulness Journey

Facing a brain cancer diagnosis is undoubtedly challenging, and embarking on a mindfulness journey can be a valuable resource for managing stress, promoting emotional well-being, and enhancing your overall quality of life. Here, we'll explore how to initiate your mindfulness practice as a brain cancer patient with a focus on setting realistic expectations, creating a quiet and comfortable space, and introducing basic mindfulness techniques for beginners.

Setting Realistic Expectations

Setting realistic mindfulness expectations as a brain cancer patient is essential to ensure that you benefit from mindfulness practices without undue pressure or disappointment. Mindfulness can be a valuable tool in coping with the challenges of brain cancer, but it's important to approach it with a practical mindset. Here are some tips for setting realistic mindfulness expectations:

1. **Understand That Mindfulness Is a Skill**: Mindfulness is not a quick fix or a one-time solution. It is a skill that requires practice and patience. Just like any other skill, it may take time to see noticeable benefits.

2. **Start Slowly**: As a brain cancer patient, you may experience physical and cognitive challenges. Begin with short, manageable mindfulness sessions. Even a few minutes a day can be beneficial. Gradually increase the duration as you become more comfortable.

3. **Be Kind to Yourself**: Mindfulness encourages self-compassion. Remember that it's okay to have wandering thoughts or moments of restlessness during your practice. Don't judge yourself for these experiences; instead, gently bring your focus back to the present.

4. **Adapt to Your Needs**: Understand that your needs may change from day to day. Some days, you may feel more energetic

and focused, while other days, you may be fatigued or in discomfort. Modify your mindfulness practice to accommodate your current state and needs.

5. **Set Realistic Goals**: Rather than expecting dramatic changes, set realistic goals for your mindfulness practice. These goals might include reducing stress, improving sleep, or simply finding moments of peace amidst the challenges of your treatment.

6. **Incorporate Mindfulness into Daily Life**: Mindfulness isn't limited to formal meditation sessions. You can incorporate it into your daily life by practicing mindfulness while eating, walking, or engaging in other routine activities. This

can make it more accessible and integrated into your life.

7. **Seek Guidance**: Consider working with a mindfulness instructor or therapist who has experience working with cancer patients. They can tailor mindfulness practices to your unique needs and help you navigate any emotional challenges that may arise.

8. **Use Mindfulness for Pain and Symptom Management**: Mindfulness can be a valuable tool for managing pain, anxiety, and other symptoms associated with brain cancer and its treatment. Set expectations for how you can use mindfulness to alleviate these specific challenges.

9. **Celebrate Small Victories**: Recognize and celebrate the small achievements and moments of clarity or peace that you experience during your mindfulness practice. These positive experiences can be motivating and reinforcing.

10. **Stay Patient and Persistent**: Consistency is key to mindfulness. Understand that it may take time to fully experience the benefits. Continue to practice regularly and stay persistent in your effort.

11. **Adapt as Needed**: Be willing to adapt your mindfulness practice as your condition and needs change throughout your cancer journey. What works for you now may need to be adjusted later.

By setting realistic expectations for your mindfulness practice as a brain cancer patient, you can experience the benefits of mindfulness while reducing any undue pressure or frustration. Remember that mindfulness is a personal journey, and its effectiveness may vary from one individual to another. Your practice is about finding what works best for you and supporting your well-being during your cancer treatment.

Creating a Quiet and Comfortable Space

Creating a quiet and comfortable space for mindfulness as a brain cancer patient can significantly enhance your practice and overall well-being. Your mindfulness space should be a sanctuary where you can find peace, relaxation, and a sense of calm. Here are some tips for creating a mindful space tailored to your unique needs:

1. Choose a Quiet Location:

- Select a quiet area in your home where you can practice mindfulness without being disturbed. Consider a room with minimal traffic or noise, such as a bedroom or a corner of a living room.

2. Minimal Distractions:

- Remove or minimize distractions. Ensure that your space is clutter-free, and put away any items that might distract you during your practice.

3. Comfortable Seating:

- Invest in a comfortable chair, cushion, or mat to sit on. Choose a seating option that accommodates your physical needs, taking into account any limitations due to your condition.

4. Personalize the Space:

- Decorate the space with items that bring you comfort and joy. These could include photos, artwork, or items with sentimental value. Create an environment that uplifts your spirit.

5. Soft Lighting:

- Use soft, diffused lighting to create a serene atmosphere. Consider using lamps with warm, soothing tones rather than harsh, bright overhead lights.

6. Peaceful Colors:

- Choose calming and soothing colors for your space. Soft blues, greens, or earthy tones can help create a tranquil atmosphere.

7. Nature Connection:

- If possible, position your mindfulness space near a window with a view of nature. Being able to gaze at trees, plants, or the sky can enhance your sense of tranquility.

8. Temperature Control:

- Ensure that the room is at a comfortable temperature. You might want to have a soft blanket or shawl nearby in case you get chilly during your practice.

9. Soundscapes or Silence:

- You can incorporate soothing background sounds, such as nature sounds or gentle music, to create a calming ambiance. Alternatively, some people prefer complete silence for their mindfulness practice.

10. Mindfulness Props: - Consider using props like a soft eye pillow, scented candles, or essential oils to enhance your sensory experience during mindfulness.

11. Accessibility: - Make sure your space is easily accessible, especially if you have physical limitations due to your condition. You should be able to reach it comfortably.

12. Create a Ritual: - Establish a routine or ritual for entering your mindful space. Lighting a candle or reciting a short affirmation can signal the beginning of your mindfulness practice.

13. Consider Safety: - If you are dealing with cognitive challenges or physical impairments, ensure that your space is safe and that you can access assistance if needed.

14. Maintain Privacy: - Make it clear to family members or caregivers that your mindfulness space is a private and sacred area where you should not be disturbed during your practice.

Your mindfulness space is a place for self-care and healing. As a brain cancer patient, it should cater to your unique needs and preferences. Regularly visit your mindful space to engage in mindfulness practices, whether it's meditation, deep breathing exercises, or simply finding a few moments of stillness. This sanctuary can provide you with solace and support throughout your journey.

Chapter 4

Breathing Techniques for Relaxation

A brain cancer diagnosis can bring with it immense stress, both physically and emotionally. To help alleviate this stress and promote relaxation, breathing techniques can be an invaluable tool for brain cancer patients. This chapter explores deep breathing for stress reduction, guided breathing exercises, and breathing techniques for pain management, offering practical ways to improve your well-being during this challenging journey.

Deep Breathing for Stress Reduction

Deep breathing can be a valuable technique for reducing stress and promoting relaxation, especially for brain cancer patients who may be dealing with various physical and emotional challenges. Here's a step-by-step guide to deep breathing for stress reduction tailored to brain cancer patients:

1. Find a Comfortable Position:

Choose a quiet and comfortable place to sit or lie down. You may want to use a chair, sit on a cushion, or lie on your back, depending on what's most comfortable for you.

2. Close Your Eyes:

Closing your eyes can help minimize external distractions and enhance your focus on the breath and relaxation.

3. Relax Your Body:

Take a moment to scan your body and consciously release any tension. Begin with your toes and work your way up to your head, relaxing each muscle group as you go.

4. Focus on Your Breath:

Breathe naturally for a few breaths, paying attention to the sensation of your breath as it enters and leaves your body.

5. Start Deep Breathing:

Begin inhaling slowly through your nose, allowing your abdomen to rise as you fill your lungs. Count to four as you inhale.

6. Hold Your Breath:

Hold your breath for a count of four.

7. Exhale Slowly:

Exhale slowly and completely through your mouth for a count of six. As you exhale, focus on releasing any tension and stress.

8. Continue the Pattern:

Continue this deep breathing pattern - inhaling for four counts, holding for four counts, and exhaling for six counts. Repeat this for several breath cycles.

9. Pay Attention to Your Breath:

As you continue deep breathing, pay close attention to the rise and fall of your abdomen with each breath. Try to make your exhalations longer than your inhalations, as this can promote relaxation.

10. Gentle Thoughts:

If your mind begins to wander or if you have thoughts related to your condition, gently acknowledge them without judgment and then return your focus to your breath.

11. Practice Regularly:

Set aside a few minutes each day to practice deep breathing. Over time, this technique can help reduce stress and promote a sense of calm and well-being.

12. Seek Guidance:

If you're new to deep breathing or if you have specific concerns related to your brain cancer or treatment, consider seeking guidance from a healthcare professional, therapist, or mindfulness instructor who can provide personalized support.

Deep breathing is a portable and accessible technique that you can use anywhere, anytime, to manage stress and promote relaxation. It's a valuable addition to your self-care routine as a brain cancer patient, helping you navigate the physical and emotional challenges you may face during your journey.

Guided Breathing Exercise

Guided breathing exercises can be a soothing and helpful practice for brain cancer patients, promoting relaxation and reducing stress. Here is a guided breathing exercise tailored for brain cancer patients:

1. Abdominal Breathing (Diaphragmatic Breathing):

This exercise focuses on deep abdominal breathing, which can help promote relaxation and reduce stress.

Instructions:

- Find a quiet and comfortable place to sit or lie down. Close your eyes if you wish.

- Place one hand on your chest and the other on your abdomen.

- Inhale slowly through your nose, allowing your abdomen to rise as you fill your lungs. Focus on the hand on your abdomen moving up while keeping the hand on your chest as still as possible.

- Exhale slowly and completely through your mouth. Feel your abdomen fall as you release the breath.

- Continue this deep, diaphragmatic breathing pattern. Inhale for a count of four, hold for a count of four, and then exhale for a count of six.

- Visualize your breath entering your body, oxygenating your cells, and exhaling any tension or stress.

- As you breathe, you can repeat calming phrases or affirmations to yourself, such as:

- "I am not alone in this journey; my loved ones are here for me."

- "My strength is inspiring, and I will draw on it."

- "It's okay to feel scared or anxious; I understand."

- "I am so loved and cherished by those around me."

- "I believe in my resilience and determination."

- "I am more than my diagnosis; I am a warrior."

- "There is hope, and I'll keep fighting for a better tomorrow."

- "I'll focus on the present moment and find peace in it."

- "I'll take deep breaths; I've got this."

- "My courage is a source of inspiration for myself and others."

- "It's okay to rest and take care of myself."

- "I'll lean on my support system; they're here to lift me up."

- "I am an incredible person, and I believe in my strength."
- "Positive thoughts and hope are my powerful allies in this journey."
- "I'll adapt and find joy in the small moments."
- "My well-being is my top priority."
- "No matter what, I am cherished and valued."
- Practice this exercise for several minutes, gradually extending the duration as you become more comfortable.

Visualization with Breath:

Visualization with breath is a relaxation technique that combines deep breathing with the power of mental imagery to promote relaxation, reduce stress, and enhance your overall well-being. Here's how to practice visualization with breath:

1. **Find a Quiet Space:** Choose a quiet and comfortable place to sit or lie down. Close your eyes and take a few moments to settle in.

2. **Deep Breathing:** Begin with a few deep breaths to relax your body. Inhale slowly through your nose, allowing your abdomen to rise, and then exhale slowly through your mouth. Repeat this a few times to calm your mind.

3. **Choose Your Visualization:** Select a peaceful and positive mental image that resonates with you. It could be a serene beach, a lush forest, a starry night sky, or any place where you feel safe and relaxed.

4. **Inhale and Envision:** As you inhale slowly through your nose, imagine yourself entering your chosen peaceful place. Picture the details – the sights, sounds, and scents. Try to engage all your senses. For example, if you're by the ocean, visualize the waves, hear them crashing, and feel the gentle breeze.

5. **Exhale and Let Go:** As you exhale through your mouth, release any tension or stress you might be feeling. Imagine exhaling

any negative energy or discomfort from your body.

6. **Repeat the Cycle:** Continue this cycle of deep breathing and visualization for several minutes. Inhale the peaceful scene and sensations, and exhale any stress or discomfort.

7. **Stay in the Moment:** Stay present in your visualization, and if your mind starts to wander, gently bring it back to your chosen peaceful place.

8. **End with Gratitude:** When you're ready to finish, take a few deep breaths and slowly open your eyes. Reflect on the relaxation and calmness you experienced during the exercise, and express gratitude for this peaceful mental escape.

Visualization with breath can be a helpful tool for managing stress, anxiety, and pain. It allows you to tap into the healing power of your imagination and breath to bring comfort and relaxation. You can use this technique as needed, whether it's during moments of stress or as part of a daily relaxation practice.

Deep breathing, guided exercise, and visualization with breath techniques are valuable resources for brain cancer patients seeking relaxation and stress reduction. These techniques are accessible, adaptable, and can significantly enhance your overall well-being during your journey. With regular practice, you can harness the healing power of your breath to support your physical and emotional needs as you navigate the complexities of brain cancer.

Chapter 5

Mindfulness Meditation Practices

Living with brain cancer can be physically and emotionally challenging. Mindfulness meditation offers valuable techniques to help patients cope with stress, reduce pain, and enhance their overall well-being. Here, we will explore mindfulness meditation practices tailored to brain cancer patients, including body scan meditation, loving-kindness meditation, walking meditation, and mindfulness of thoughts and emotions.

Body Scan Meditation

Brain cancer is a challenging and often painful journey for both the patient and their loved ones. Coping with the diagnosis, treatments, and the uncertainty that accompanies it can be mentally and physically exhausting. In such circumstances, complementary practices like body scan meditation can provide much-needed relief and support in the holistic approach to healing.

Understanding the Power of Body Scan Meditation

Body scan meditation is a mindfulness practice that involves systematically focusing on different parts of the body, from head to toe or vice versa, to promote relaxation, self-awareness, and emotional well-being. It's a deeply nurturing and therapeutic practice that can benefit brain cancer patients in several ways.

Emotional and Psychological Benefits

- Stress Reduction
- Improved Sleep
- Enhanced Emotional Regulation

Physical Benefits

- Pain Management
- Enhanced Body Awareness

Quality of Life and Coping Mechanism

- Empowerment
- Coping with Uncertainty:

How to Practice Body Scan Meditation for Brain Cancer Patients

1. **Find a Quiet and Comfortable Space:** Select a calm and distraction-free environment where you can sit or lie down. Ensure you are comfortable and well-supported.

2. **Deep Breathing:** Start by taking a few deep, calming breaths to center yourself and bring your focus to the present moment.

3. **Begin at the Head:** Gently direct your attention to the top of your head. Pay close attention to any sensations, such as warmth, tingling, or tension.

4. **Systematic Scanning:** Progressively move your focus down through your body, one area at a time. Proceed from your head to your toes or vice versa, whichever feels

more comfortable. Explore your neck, shoulders, chest, arms, abdomen, pelvis, thighs, knees, calves, ankles, and feet.

5. **Breath Synchronization**: Coordinate your breath with the scanning process. Inhale as you focus on an area and exhale as you release tension or discomfort from that area.

6. **Non-Judgmental Awareness**: Remember that this practice is about observing your body without judgment. If you encounter pain or discomfort, acknowledge it without trying to change it.

7. **Regular Practice**: Consistency is key. Set aside dedicated time for body scan meditation each day or as needed.

8. **Seek Guidance:** If you are new to meditation or require extra support, consider using guided body scan meditations available through meditation apps, websites, or with the guidance of a healthcare professional.

The Journey to Healing and Inner Peace

In the face of brain cancer, body scan meditation is a gentle yet powerful practice that can provide solace and relief to patients. It fosters emotional well-being, reduces stress, and enhances body awareness. By incorporating this meditation practice into their daily routines, patients can take an active role in their healing journey, improve their quality of life, and find moments of inner peace amid the challenges they face. This mindfulness practice complements medical treatment by nurturing not just the body but the mind and spirit as well.

Loving-Kindness Meditation

Loving-Kindness Meditation (Metta Meditation) is a beautiful and heartwarming practice that can provide solace, emotional support, and positivity to individuals facing challenging situations such as brain cancer. This meditation encourages feelings of compassion and love, not only for others but also for oneself. It's a powerful tool for promoting emotional healing and well-being. Here's a guide on how to practice Loving-Kindness Meditation for a brain cancer patient:

Preparing for Loving-Kindness Meditation

1. **Find a Quiet Space**: Select a peaceful and quiet location where you won't be disturbed during the meditation. Comfort is key.

2. **Comfortable Posture**: Sit in a comfortable position, either in a chair or on the floor, or you can even practice this meditation while lying down.

3. **Begin with Deep Breathing**: Start the meditation by taking a few deep breaths. Inhale through your nose and exhale through your mouth, gradually calming your mind and body.

The Loving-Kindness Meditation Practice

1. Send Kindness to Yourself

- Begin by focusing on yourself. Silently repeat these phrases or adapt them as you see fit: "May I be happy. May I be healthy. May I live with ease." These phrases express your wish for well-being and contentment for yourself.

- As you recite these phrases, truly feel the warmth of your own compassion and the intention behind your words. Allow yourself to be the recipient of your own love and kindness.

- Spend a few minutes in this self-focused loving-kindness meditation. Imagine the warmth and healing energy filling your entire being.

2. Extend Kindness to Loved Ones

- Shift your focus to someone close to you, perhaps a family member, friend, or caregiver who has been supporting you through your journey with brain cancer.

- Repeat the phrases, directing them toward your loved one. For example, "May you be happy. May you be healthy. May you live with ease."

- Imagine your love and compassion radiating from your heart to theirs, embracing them in a warm, healing light.

3. Offer Kindness to Neutral Individuals

- Now, turn your attention to someone you don't have strong feelings about, someone more neutral in your life. It could be a neighbor, colleague, or acquaintance.

- Send your well wishes to them with the same phrases: "May you be happy. May you be healthy. May you live with ease."

- Visualize the positive energy extending to this individual, enveloping them in love and warmth.

4. Extend Kindness to Challenging Individuals

- This step can be the most challenging but also the most transformative.

Think of someone you may have conflicts or difficulties with, and direct the phrases of loving-kindness toward them.

- With an open heart, wish them happiness, health, and ease: "May you be happy. May you be healthy. May you live with ease."

- As you do this, envision the healing energy softening any tension or animosity between you and this person.

5. Widen the Circle of Compassion

- Expand your circle of compassion to include all beings, not just those in your immediate life. Visualize a world filled with individuals experiencing happiness, health, and ease.

- Say the loving-kindness phrases once more: "May all beings be happy. May all beings be healthy. May all beings live with ease."

- Imagine your love and compassion spreading out to encompass everyone, and visualize a world transformed by kindness and positivity.

Ending the Meditation

1. **Gentle Return:** Gradually bring your awareness back to the room, the present moment, and your own breath.

2. **Reflect:** Take a moment to reflect on the meditation and the feelings of love and compassion it has cultivated.

3. **Daily Practice:** Loving-Kindness Meditation can be practiced daily to nurture and strengthen feelings of love and kindness within yourself, fostering emotional well-being and resilience in the face of adversity.

Loving-Kindness Meditation can serve as a powerful emotional anchor for brain cancer patients, helping them navigate their journey with a heart full of compassion and resilience. It promotes self-love, positive relationships, and an empathetic connection to others, all of which are crucial elements in the healing process.

Walking Meditation

Walking meditation is a mindful practice that can be particularly beneficial for brain cancer patients. It offers a way to engage with the world and your own body in a gentle and contemplative manner. Here's a guide on how to practice walking meditation for a brain cancer patient:

Preparing for Walking Meditation

1. **Choose a Safe and Quiet Location**: Find a safe, peaceful area for your walking meditation. This can be indoors or outdoors, depending on your preference and mobility.

2. **Comfortable Attire**: Wear comfortable clothing and shoes. Ensure you're dressed appropriately for the weather if you're doing your meditation outdoors.

3. **Set an Intention**: Before you start, set an intention for your walking meditation. It could be focused on finding peace, reducing stress, or simply enjoying the present moment.

The Walking Meditation Practice

1. **Stand Still**: Begin by standing still for a few moments. Close your eyes if you feel comfortable, and take a few deep breaths. Allow yourself to arrive fully in the present moment.

2. **Awareness of Posture**: As you start walking, become aware of your posture. Stand up straight, with your head held high but relaxed, and your arms hanging naturally by your sides.

3. **Mindful Steps**: Begin to walk slowly, taking each step with intention and mindfulness. Focus on the sensation of your feet lifting off the ground, moving through the air, and making contact with the earth.

4. **Breath Awareness**: Pay attention to your breath as you walk. Sync your breathing with your steps, taking a deep inhale for a certain number of steps and then exhaling for the same number of steps.

5. **Mindful Steps**: With each step, become fully present in the act of walking. Notice how your feet feel as they touch the ground. Feel the earth beneath you supporting your steps.

6. **Sensory Awareness**: Engage your senses as you walk. Pay attention to the sounds around you, the feeling of the air on your skin, and any scents in the environment.

7. **Focus on the Moment**: Gently let go of any thoughts about the past or worries about the future. Keep your attention on the here and now.

8. **Walking Path**: You can walk in a straight line, in a circle, or follow any path you choose. The length of your

walk is not as important as the quality of your presence.

9. **Turning and Continuing**: If you reach the end of your walking path, stop, take a breath, and turn mindfully. Continue walking in the opposite direction, maintaining your awareness.

10. **Gratitude and Reflection**: As you walk, reflect on things you're grateful for or positive aspects of your life. Gratitude can be a powerful emotional tool.

11. **Coping and Healing**: If you're using walking meditation as part of your healing journey, you can also focus your attention on sending positive energy to the affected parts of your

body. Imagine healing light and positive intentions being directed toward those areas.

12.   **Ending the Meditation**: When you're ready to end your walking meditation, come to a stop. Take a moment to stand still and appreciate the experience. Notice how you feel after the practice.

Consistency and Adaptation

Walking meditation can be adapted to your specific needs and capabilities. If you have limited mobility, you can practice mindful walking in a smaller space or even in place. The key is to be fully present, move with intention, and engage your senses and breath.

Consistency is valuable, so aim to make walking meditation a regular practice. It can serve as a soothing and grounding activity for brain cancer patients, offering a way to connect with the world and with yourself, and fostering a sense of inner peace and healing.

Mindfulness of Thoughts and Emotions

Mindfulness of thoughts and emotions is a valuable practice for brain cancer patients. This mindfulness technique can help patients cope with the emotional challenges and uncertainties that often come with the diagnosis and treatment of such a serious illness. Here's a guide on how to practice mindfulness of thoughts and emotions:

Preparing for Mindfulness of Thoughts and Emotions

1. **Find a Quiet and Comfortable Space:** Start by selecting a peaceful and comfortable place where you can sit or lie down. It should be a space where you feel safe and can focus without distractions.

2. **Set an Intention:** Begin your practice by setting an intention. What would you like to achieve from this mindfulness session? It could be to find peace, reduce anxiety, or simply to better understand your thoughts and emotions.

3. **Comfortable Posture**: Sit or lie down in a comfortable position. You can use a cushion or chair to support your posture. Ensure that you're at ease and well-supported.

4. **Begin with Deep Breathing**: Start the mindfulness practice with several deep breaths. Inhale slowly through your nose and exhale through your mouth, gradually calming your mind and body.

The Mindfulness of Thoughts and Emotions Practice

1. **Thought Observation**: Close your eyes, and turn your attention to your thoughts. Allow your thoughts to flow naturally, and observe them without judgment. Don't try to change or suppress them.

2. **Emotion Awareness**: As you observe your thoughts, pay attention to the emotions that accompany them. Notice how different thoughts elicit different emotional responses.

3. **Name the Emotions**: When you identify an emotion, name it silently. For example, if you're feeling anxious, say to yourself, "This is anxiety." Labeling the emotion can create a sense of distance and objectivity.

4. **Breathe Through Emotions**: As you continue to observe your thoughts and emotions, use your breath as an anchor. Whenever you encounter a strong or distressing emotion, take a few deep breaths. Inhale through your nose, hold

for a moment, and then exhale slowly through your mouth. This can help you stay grounded.

5. **Non-Judgmental Observation:** Remember that the goal is not to judge yourself for your thoughts or emotions. Instead, practice non-judgmental observation. Accept what arises without attaching any value to it.

6. **Letting Go**: When you're ready, imagine placing your thoughts and emotions on a metaphorical leaf in a gently flowing stream. Watch them drift away as you release them, knowing that they don't define you.

7. **Return to the Present**: If your mind starts to wander into the past or future, gently bring it back to the present moment. Focus on your breath, the sensations in your body, or the sounds in your environment.

8. **Acceptance and Self-Compassion:** Throughout the practice, maintain a sense of self-compassion and acceptance. Recognize that it's okay to have these thoughts and emotions, and that they are part of the human experience.

9. **Duration**: You can practice mindfulness of thoughts and emotions for as long as you feel comfortable. Starting with 10-15 minutes and gradually increasing the duration can be beneficial.

10. **Reflection**: After your mindfulness session, take a moment to reflect on your experience. What did you observe about your thoughts and emotions? How do you feel now compared to when you started the practice?

Integration and Consistency

Mindfulness of thoughts and emotions is a practice that can be integrated into your daily life. By regularly setting aside time to observe your thoughts and emotions without judgment, you can develop a deeper understanding of your inner world and cultivate emotional resilience. It can be particularly valuable for brain cancer patients as it offers a way to process the complex emotions and thoughts that arise during their journey.

As a brain cancer patient, mindfulness meditation practices can offer solace, empowerment, and emotional support. These techniques can be adapted to your unique needs and abilities, providing you with valuable tools to navigate the challenges of your condition while promoting relaxation and well-being.

Progressive Muscle Relaxation

Progressive Muscle Relaxation (PMR) can be a helpful technique for brain cancer patients to reduce stress, ease physical discomfort, and promote relaxation. Given the unique challenges faced by brain cancer patients, it's essential to adapt PMR to their specific needs. Here's a modified version of PMR tailored for brain cancer patients:

1. Find a Quiet Space: Begin by choosing a quiet and comfortable space where you won't be disturbed.

2. Comfortable Position: Sit or lie down in a comfortable position. You can use pillows or blankets for added comfort and support.

3. Focus on Breathing: Close your eyes and take a few deep, calming breaths to center yourself. Inhale deeply through your nose and exhale slowly through your mouth.

4. Mindful Awareness: Bring your attention to the present moment, acknowledging any physical discomfort or tension you might be experiencing. This mindfulness allows you to identify areas of the body that need relaxation.

5. Gentle Tension and Release: Given the potential physical limitations, you may not be able to tense and release muscles as vigorously as in traditional PMR. Instead, focus on gentle, subtle movements. For example:

- Wiggle your toes and fingers to improve circulation and promote a sense of connection with your body.

- Imagine a warm, soothing sensation washing over your head and neck, relaxing any tension.

6. Guided Visualization: Incorporate guided visualization to replace traditional muscle tension and relaxation. Visualize a wave of calm and healing energy flowing through your body, focusing on areas affected by your condition.

7. Mindful Breathing: Continue to focus on your breath. Inhale tranquility and exhale any stress or discomfort. Imagine each breath providing relief and comfort.

8. Body Scanning: Gradually scan your body from head to toe. Pay attention to any areas where you feel discomfort or tension. Imagine these areas softening and relaxing as you breathe.

9. Affirmations: Incorporate positive affirmations related to your condition, such as "I am resilient," "I am surrounded by love and support," or any other affirmations that resonate with you.

10. Gratitude: Express gratitude for your body and its resilience. Focus on the parts of your body that are healthy and functioning well.

11. Slowly Open Your Eyes: When you're ready, open your eyes and reorient yourself to the present moment. Take a few moments to reflect on the sense of calm and relaxation you've cultivated.

Customizing PMR for brain cancer patients with gentle movements, visualization, and mindfulness can provide comfort and relaxation while taking into consideration any physical limitations or discomfort associated with the condition. As always, consult with healthcare professionals or therapists for guidance and to ensure that this practice aligns with your specific needs and medical situation.

Chapter 6

Affirmations

Affirmations can be a powerful tool for brain cancer patients to cultivate a positive mindset, boost resilience, and promote emotional well-being. Here are some affirmations tailored to the unique challenges and experiences of brain cancer patients:

1. "I am stronger than my diagnosis. I can overcome the challenges that come my way."

2. "My body has incredible healing abilities, and I am supporting it every day."

3.   "I am surrounded by a supportive and loving network of friends and family."

4.   "I embrace each day with hope, gratitude, and a positive attitude."

5.   "I trust my medical team and the treatment plan they have developed for me."

6.   "I am not defined by my illness. I am defined by my strength, resilience, and character."

7.   "I am in control of my thoughts and emotions, and I choose positivity and hope."

8.   "Every day, I am getting closer to healing and recovery."

9.   "I am a survivor, and I am determined to live a meaningful and fulfilling life."

10.   "I am a source of inspiration to others who are facing their own challenges."

11.   "I have the inner strength to face uncertainty and fear with courage and grace."

12.   "I am grateful for the small joys and moments of beauty that each day brings."

13.   "I am at peace with the present moment and accept it with an open heart."

14.   "I am deserving of self-compassion and self-care during this journey."

15.   "I believe in my body's ability to heal, and I am doing everything I can to support it."

16.   "I am resilient, and I can find moments of joy even in difficult times."

17.   "I am surrounded by the healing power of love, hope, and positive energy."

18.   "I am focused on the present, taking one step at a time toward a brighter future."

19.   "I am grateful for the medical advancements and support available to me."

20.   "I am a beacon of hope, showing others that a positive outlook can make a significant difference."

21.   "I am living each day with purpose and intention, making the most of every moment."

22. "I am a warrior, and my battle with brain cancer will only make me stronger."

23. "I am connected to the healing energy of the universe, which supports my well-being."

24. "I trust my inner wisdom to guide me through the challenges I face."

25. "I am grateful for the lessons that my journey with brain cancer is teaching me."

26. "I have the courage to face uncertainty with grace and resilience."

27. "I am surrounded by the beauty of life, even in the midst of difficulty."

28. "I am a beacon of strength and hope, inspiring those around me."

29. "I believe in the power of a positive mindset to aid in my healing."

30. "I am not alone in this journey; I am part of a community that understands and supports me."

31. "I am embracing self-care as an essential part of my healing journey."

32. "I am finding comfort in the love and care of my support network."

33. "I am resilient and adaptable, able to adjust to the challenges that arise."

34. "I am letting go of fear and embracing the peace that comes with acceptance."

35. "I am grateful for the gift of life, and I cherish each moment."

36. "I am open to new possibilities and opportunities that may arise on this path."

37.   "I am a source of inspiration, reminding others of the strength that lies within."

38.   "I am focusing on the things I can control and letting go of what I cannot."

39.   "I am proud of my ability to endure and persevere through the toughest times."

40.   "I am surrounded by love, which is a powerful force for healing."

Use these affirmations as a daily practice, repeating them to yourself with sincerity and belief. You can customize and create your own affirmations that resonate most with your experiences and aspirations. Affirmations can be a valuable part of a holistic approach to healing and emotional well-being during your journey with brain cancer.

Chapter 7

Mindful Eating and Nutrition

For cancer patients, nutrition plays a crucial role in supporting health and well-being during and after treatment. Particularly for brain cancer patients, mindful eating can be a valuable tool to enhance brain health, manage side effects of treatment, and promote overall well-being. In this guide, we'll explore the relationship between diet and brain health, mindful eating practices, and how to nourish your body effectively during cancer treatment.

The Relationship Between Diet and Brain Health

The relationship between diet and brain health is crucial, especially for individuals dealing with brain cancer. A well-balanced and nutritious diet can play a significant role in supporting overall health and potentially improving the quality of life for brain cancer patients. Here's a discussion on the topic, taking into consideration the unique needs and challenges that these patients face:

Nutritional Considerations for Brain Cancer Patients

1. Caloric and Protein Requirements: Brain cancer patients often experience increased calorie and protein requirements due to the metabolic demands of the disease and its treatment. Adequate protein intake is essential for maintaining and repairing tissues.

2. Hydration: Dehydration is a common concern, as brain cancer patients may experience symptoms like nausea, vomiting, and cognitive changes. Staying well-hydrated is vital for cognitive function and overall well-being.

3. Nutrient-Dense Foods: Focus on nutrient-dense foods such as fruits, vegetables, lean proteins, whole grains, and healthy fats. These foods provide essential vitamins, minerals, and antioxidants that support the immune system and overall health.

4. Omega-3 Fatty Acids: Omega-3 fatty acids, found in fatty fish like salmon and walnuts, have anti-inflammatory properties and may help reduce inflammation and support brain health.

5. Antioxidants: Antioxidant-rich foods like berries, leafy greens, and dark chocolate can help protect brain cells from damage and promote overall well-being.

6. Small, Frequent Meals: Some brain cancer patients may struggle with appetite changes or digestive issues. Eating smaller, frequent meals can be easier to manage and ensure a steady supply of nutrients.

7. **Limiting Processed Foods:** Highly processed and sugary foods can lead to energy spikes and crashes. Reducing these in the diet can help stabilize energy levels and prevent unhealthy weight fluctuations.

8. **Adapting to Symptoms:** Brain cancer symptoms and treatments can result in specific dietary challenges, such as difficulty swallowing or taste changes. Consulting with a dietitian or nutritionist can help tailor the diet to address these issues.

9. **Consult with Healthcare Team:** It's essential for brain cancer patients to consult with their healthcare team, including a dietitian or nutritionist, to create a personalized nutrition plan that addresses their specific needs and treatment-related

challenges.

10. Maintain Healthy Weight: Maintaining a healthy weight is essential for overall health and can help the body better cope with the physical and emotional challenges associated with brain cancer.

The Role of Diet in Brain Health

The brain requires a constant supply of nutrients and energy to function optimally. A diet rich in essential nutrients can support cognitive function, mood stability, and overall brain health. For brain cancer patients, this is especially important due to the potential impact of the disease and its treatments on cognitive and emotional well-being.

- **Cognitive Function:** Proper nutrition can help preserve cognitive function, which is often affected in brain cancer patients. Nutrients like antioxidants, omega-3 fatty acids, and vitamins support brain health and may contribute to improved cognitive function.

- **Mood and Emotional Well-being:** A balanced diet can have a significant impact on mood and emotional well-being. Consuming nutrient-dense foods and maintaining stable blood sugar levels can help reduce mood swings and feelings of anxiety or depression.

- **Supporting Immune Function:** Brain cancer patients may have compromised immune systems due to the disease or its treatment. Proper nutrition can bolster the immune system and support the body's natural defenses.

- **Reducing Inflammation:** Chronic inflammation is linked to various health issues, including cancer. An anti-inflammatory diet, rich in whole foods and antioxidants, can help reduce inflammation and promote brain health.

- **Reducing Side Effects:** Nutritional strategies can help mitigate some of the side effects of cancer treatments, such as nausea, vomiting, and fatigue. Specialized diets can be designed to alleviate these symptoms.

Diet plays a critical role in the overall well-being and quality of life of brain cancer patients. A balanced and nutritious diet can help support cognitive function, emotional well-being, and immune function. It can also help manage the side effects of cancer treatments. Consulting with a healthcare team and a registered dietitian is crucial for creating a personalized nutrition plan that addresses the specific needs and challenges of each patient. By focusing on nourishing the body and brain, brain cancer patients can enhance their overall health and well-being during their journey.

Mindful Eating Practices

Mindful eating is a beneficial practice for brain cancer patients, as it can help improve their overall well-being and quality of life. Here are some mindful eating practices tailored to the specific needs and challenges that brain cancer patients may face:

1. Eating Environment

- **Choose a Peaceful Setting**: Opt for a quiet and pleasant environment for meals. Reducing distractions can help you focus on your food.

- **Use Calming Elements**: Incorporate elements that promote relaxation, such as soft music, candles, or a table setting that brings you joy.

- **Comfortable Seating**: Make sure you're seated in a comfortable and supportive chair. This is especially important if you're experiencing fatigue or discomfort.

2. Gratitude and Intention

- **Express Gratitude**: Begin your meal with a moment of gratitude. Reflect on the food in front of you and appreciate it. This simple practice can foster a positive mindset.

- **Set an Intention**: Before you start eating, set an intention for the meal. This could be to nourish your body, enjoy the flavors, or simply to savor the experience.

3. Mindful Observation

- **Observe Your Food**: Take a moment to observe your meal with all your senses. Notice the colors, textures, and aromas of the food. Engage your senses fully.

- **Appreciate the Journey**: Consider the journey of the food, from its source to your plate. This practice can deepen your connection to the food.

4. Mindful Eating

- **Eat Slowly**: Consciously take your time with each bite. Savor the flavors, and chew your food thoroughly. Eating slowly promotes digestion and allows you to better enjoy your meal.

- **Put Down Utensils**: Between bites, put down your fork or spoon. This encourages a mindful pause and prevents rushing through your meal.

- **Tune In to Hunger Cues**: Pay attention to your body's hunger and fullness signals. Eat until you're comfortably satisfied, not overly full.

5. Managing Symptoms

- **Adapt to Symptoms**: Brain cancer and its treatment can cause symptoms like nausea, changes in taste, or difficulty swallowing. It's important to adapt your meals to manage these symptoms. Choose softer or blander foods if necessary.

- **Stay Hydrated**: Adequate hydration is vital. Sip water or other hydrating beverages between bites to ensure you stay well-hydrated, especially if treatment causes dry mouth.

- **Small, Frequent Meals**: If you struggle with appetite changes or digestive issues, consider eating smaller, more frequent meals throughout the day.

6. Emotional Awareness

- **Check-In with Emotions**: Take a moment to check in with your emotional state before, during, and after a meal. Mindful eating can help you better understand the connection between your emotions and eating habits.

- **Non-Judgmental Awareness**: Approach your emotions and thoughts about food with non-judgmental awareness. Accept how you feel without self-criticism.

7. Mindful Portion Control

- **Portion Size**: Be mindful of portion sizes. Use smaller plates or bowls to help with portion control. This can be particularly beneficial if you're managing weight changes.

8. Mindful Reflection

- **Reflect After Eating**: After you finish your meal, reflect on the experience. How did it make you feel physically and emotionally? What did you enjoy most about the meal?

- **Gratitude:** Once again, express gratitude for the nourishment you've received.

Mindful eating practices can enhance the overall experience of meals, improve digestion, and foster a positive relationship with food. They can also help brain cancer patients manage the specific challenges that come with their condition and its treatment. By approaching meals with mindfulness, you can create a sense of calm and nourishment that contributes to your well-being during your journey.

Nourishing Your Body During Treatment

Nourishing your body during brain cancer treatment is crucial to support your health, maintain strength, and manage potential side effects. Here are some guidelines to help you provide your body with the best possible nutrition during this challenging time:

1. Work with a Registered Dietitian

Collaborate with a registered dietitian who specializes in oncology nutrition. They can create a personalized nutrition plan that addresses your specific needs, including treatment side effects and any dietary restrictions.

2. Opt for Nutrient-Dense Foods

Focus on foods that provide the most nutrients for your body:

- **Fruits and Vegetables:** Choose a variety of colorful fruits and vegetables to supply essential vitamins, minerals, and antioxidants that support your immune system.

- **Lean Proteins:** Include lean protein sources like poultry, fish, lean meats, beans, and tofu to help repair tissues and maintain muscle mass.

- **Whole Grains:** Opt for whole grains like brown rice, quinoa, and whole wheat to provide complex carbohydrates for sustained energy.

- **Healthy Fats:** Incorporate sources of healthy fats like avocados, nuts, seeds, and olive oil. These fats support brain health and overall well-being.

3. Stay Hydrated

Dehydration can be a common issue during cancer treatment. Ensure you're staying well-hydrated by sipping water throughout the day. If you have trouble with water due to taste changes, consider adding a splash of lemon or using a straw to make drinking more comfortable.

4. Small, Frequent Meals

Rather than traditional three meals a day, consider eating smaller, more frequent meals. This can help manage appetite changes, reduce digestive discomfort, and ensure a steady supply of nutrients.

5. Adapt to Symptoms and Side Effects

Brain cancer treatment often brings side effects that can affect your appetite and ability to eat. Adapt your diet to manage these symptoms:

- **Nausea and Vomiting**: Opt for bland, easily digestible foods. Ginger and peppermint tea can help alleviate nausea.

- **Taste Changes**: Experiment with different flavors and spices. Some people find sour or spicy foods more appealing during treatment.

- **Dry Mouth**: Keep your mouth moist by sipping water, sucking on ice chips, or using sugar-free candies or gum.

- **Swallowing Difficulty**: Choose softer foods like mashed potatoes, smoothies, and soups. You can also try pureed or blended foods.

6. Supplements

Talk to your healthcare team about the need for supplements. Depending on your diet and specific needs, you may require nutritional supplements, such as vitamins, minerals, or protein shakes.

7. Emotional Support

Eating can be emotional during cancer treatment. Reach out to a therapist, support group, or counselor to help you cope with the psychological aspects of managing your diet.

8. Listen to Your Body

Pay attention to your body's signals. If you're not hungry or experiencing digestive discomfort, it's okay to eat less or skip a meal. Rest when you need to, and practice self-compassion throughout your journey.

9. Maintain a Positive Outlook

A positive attitude can play a role in healing. Embrace a mindset that views food as nourishment for your body and a vital component of your healing process.

10. Communicate with Your Healthcare Team

Regularly communicate with your healthcare team about any changes in your appetite, weight, or side effects. They can adjust your treatment plan or provide additional support as needed.

Nourishing your body during brain cancer treatment is a critical aspect of your overall care. By working closely with healthcare professionals, adapting to your specific challenges, and focusing on nutrient-dense foods, you can provide your body with the support it needs to endure and recover from treatment.

Chapter 8

Techniques for Dealing with Treatment Side Effects

Brain cancer treatments, such as surgery, radiation therapy, and chemotherapy, often come with various side effects that can be physically and emotionally challenging. Here are some techniques and strategies to help brain cancer patients cope with and manage these treatment side effects:

1. Nausea and Vomiting

- **Anti-Nausea Medications**: Work closely with your healthcare team to find the most suitable anti-nausea medications to prevent or relieve nausea and vomiting.

- **Ginger and Peppermint**: Try ginger or peppermint tea, candies, or supplements, as these natural remedies can help alleviate nausea.

- **Dietary Changes**: Opt for bland, easily digestible foods like rice, bananas, and applesauce. Small, frequent meals can also help prevent nausea.

2. Fatigue

- **Rest and Sleep**: Prioritize rest and ensure you're getting enough sleep. Short naps during the day can be helpful, but try to maintain a regular sleep schedule.

- **Physical Activity**: Engage in gentle physical activities like walking or yoga to boost energy levels and improve mood.

- **Pacing Yourself**: Learn to pace your activities and take breaks when needed to conserve energy.

3. Cognitive Changes (Chemo Brain)

- **Mental Exercises**: Engage in cognitive exercises like puzzles, memory games, or reading to help maintain mental function.

- **Mindfulness and Meditation**: Mindfulness practices can help improve focus and cognitive function.

- **Simplify Tasks**: Break tasks into smaller, manageable steps to avoid feeling overwhelmed.

4. Taste Changes

- **Experiment with Flavors**: Try foods with different flavors, temperatures, or textures to see what appeals to your changing taste buds.

- **Sour and Spicy Foods**: Some patients find sour or spicy foods more palatable when experiencing taste changes.

- **Food Presentation**: Make your meals visually appealing to stimulate your appetite.

5. Dry Mouth

- **Oral Hygiene**: Maintain good oral hygiene to prevent dental problems. Use mouthwashes designed for dry mouth.

- **Hydration**: Sip water frequently to keep your mouth moist.

- **Sugar-Free Lozenges and Gum**: Sugar-free candies or gum can help stimulate saliva production.

6. Pain and Discomfort

- **Pain Medications**: Work with your healthcare team to manage and alleviate pain using appropriate medications.

- **Heat and Cold Therapy**: Heat or cold packs can be helpful for pain relief, depending on the type of pain.

- **Relaxation Techniques**: Practices like deep breathing and progressive muscle relaxation can reduce pain-related tension.

7. Emotional Support

- **Therapy and Counseling**: Seek support from a therapist or counselor to cope with emotional challenges and anxiety.

- **Support Groups**: Join a support group for brain cancer patients to share experiences and receive emotional support from those who understand.

- **Express Yourself**: Share your feelings with loved ones. Open and honest communication can help alleviate emotional distress.

8. Physical Activity

- **Gentle Exercise**: Engage in light physical activity like walking, stretching, or yoga, as it can help with overall well-being and mood.

- **Consult with a Physical Therapist**: If you experience physical limitations, consider working with a physical therapist to address mobility and strength issues.

9. Dietary Modifications

- **Collaborate with a Dietitian**: A registered dietitian can create a personalized nutrition plan to address dietary changes and challenges.

- **Small, Frequent Meals**: If appetite or digestive issues are a concern, consider eating smaller, more frequent meals.

10. Communicate with Your Healthcare Team

- **Regular Updates**: Maintain open communication with your healthcare team about any side effects, changes in your condition, or any concerns you have.

- **Medication Adjustments:** If side effects are severe or debilitating, your healthcare team can adjust your treatment plan or medications accordingly.

Coping with brain cancer treatment side effects can be challenging, but with the right strategies and support, patients can minimize discomfort and maintain a better quality of life. Open and honest communication with your healthcare team is essential to address your specific needs and ensure the most effective treatment and symptom management.

Guided Imagery for Comfort

Guided imagery is a powerful relaxation technique that can provide comfort and emotional support for brain cancer patients. It involves using your imagination to create calming, positive mental images that promote relaxation and well-being. Here's a guided imagery script specifically designed for comfort and relaxation:

Before you begin, find a quiet and comfortable place to sit or lie down. Close your eyes and take a few deep breaths to help you relax.

Introduction:

- Imagine yourself in a peaceful and serene place, free from worries and pain.

- Picture a place that brings you a sense of comfort and security. It could be a favorite spot from your past or an entirely imaginary place of your creation.

- As you go through this guided imagery, remember that you are in control, and you can choose to modify the images and scenes to suit your preferences.

The Beach Visualization:

- Picture yourself on a beautiful, tranquil beach. Feel the warm sand underneath you, providing a soft, comforting embrace.

The Sound of Waves:

- Imagine the soothing sound of gentle waves rolling in and out. With each wave, feel tension and discomfort leaving your body.

Warmth and Light:

- Envision the sun above you, radiating warmth and comfort. Feel its gentle rays on your skin, healing and revitalizing.

The Ocean Breeze:

- As you breathe in, imagine the fresh, salty breeze from the ocean filling your lungs. With each exhale, release any stress, fear, or pain.

Nature's Healing:

- Picture the water's edge, where the waves kiss the shore. Visualize the water as a source of healing energy, washing over you and soothing any discomfort.

Surrounded by Loved Ones:

- Imagine the presence of loved ones or supportive figures around you on this beach. They offer you love, warmth, and understanding. You are not alone.

Comforting Colors:

- Visualize the colors of the beach around you - the blue of the ocean, the golden sand, and the vibrant green of the palm trees. Let these colors fill you with peace and comfort.

Safe Haven:

- You are in a safe place, free from pain and worry. Your body and mind are at ease, allowing you to heal and find comfort.

Progressive Relaxation:

- As you lie on the beach, scan your body from head to toe, releasing any tension or discomfort you find. With each breath, let go of any tightness and pain.

Floating on Calm Waters:

- Now, imagine yourself floating on the gentle waves of the ocean. As you drift on the water, any discomfort or fear drifts away from you.

Restorative Healing:

- The water embraces you with its healing energy. Feel it washing away any negativity, leaving you refreshed and comforted.

Closing:

- Take a few moments to relish this sense of comfort and healing. You can return to this peaceful place whenever you need comfort and relaxation.

When you're ready, gently bring your awareness back to the present moment. Open your eyes and carry this sense of comfort with you throughout the day.

Guided imagery can be a valuable tool for brain cancer patients to find comfort, reduce stress, and promote overall well-being. It allows you to create a mental safe haven where you can find solace and peace during your challenging journey.

Managing pain and discomfort as a brain cancer patient requires a combination of techniques, including mindfulness, practical strategies for treatment side effects, and guided imagery for comfort. By incorporating these approaches into your daily life, you can enhance your well-being and find relief in the midst of your cancer journey. Always consult with your healthcare team to ensure that your chosen methods align with your specific treatment plan and needs.

Chapter 9

Coping with Emotional Challenges

Living with brain cancer can bring a range of emotional challenges, from anxiety and depression to the quest for joy and gratitude in each moment. Coping with these emotions is essential for maintaining emotional well-being during your cancer journey. In this chapter, we will explore strategies to address anxiety and depression, discover moments of joy and gratitude, and use mindfulness to improve sleep.

Addressing Anxiety and Depression

To address anxiety and depression for a brain cancer patient, you must understand that these emotional challenges are common and valid responses to the diagnosis and treatment process. As you navigate this difficult journey, consider the following strategies to help you cope with anxiety and depression:

1. **Seek Professional Support**: It's essential to reach out to mental health professionals who specialize in working with individuals facing chronic illness. Psychologists or psychiatrists can provide therapeutic interventions tailored to your specific needs.

2. **Therapy:** Individual or group therapy sessions offer a safe and supportive environment for exploring and managing the emotional aspects of living with brain cancer. Talking with a trained therapist can help you process your feelings and develop coping strategies.

3. **Medication:** In some cases, your healthcare team may recommend medication to manage the symptoms of anxiety and depression. Always consult with a qualified medical professional who can prescribe and monitor medication when necessary.

4. **Connect with Support Networks:** Joining brain cancer support groups, whether in-person or online, can provide a sense of

community and emotional support. You'll find others who understand your journey and can offer valuable insights and encouragement.

5. **Practice Mindfulness and Meditation:** Mindfulness meditation can be a powerful tool for managing your emotional well-being. Through mindfulness, you can learn to be present in the moment, accept your emotions without judgment, and effectively manage stress.

6. **Engage in Regular Exercise:** Physical activity has been proven to have a positive impact on mood. Even gentle exercises like walking or yoga can help reduce symptoms of anxiety and

depression while promoting overall well-being.

7. **Cognitive-Behavioral Therapy (CBT)**: This type of therapy can help you identify and reframe negative thought patterns that contribute to anxiety and depression. With the guidance of a trained therapist, you can work on changing unhelpful thinking habits.

8. **Prioritize Nutrition and Sleep**: Your emotional well-being is closely connected to your physical health. A balanced diet and quality sleep are essential. Nutrient-rich foods can support your mood, and ensuring you get enough rest is crucial for managing anxiety and depression.

9. **Learn Coping Strategies**: Explore stress management techniques like deep breathing, progressive muscle relaxation, and journaling. These methods can help you better cope with the emotional challenges you're facing.

10. **Practice Self-Compassion**: Remember to be kind to yourself. Prioritize self-care and acknowledge the unique challenges you're experiencing. Self-compassion can significantly improve your emotional well-being.

11. **Keep Communication Open**: Effective communication between you, your family, and your healthcare team is crucial. By discussing your emotional concerns openly, you can ensure that

your treatment and support are aligned with your specific needs.

12. **End-of-Life Planning and Palliative Care**: In cases where brain cancer is advanced, addressing end-of-life care and planning can provide emotional relief. Open discussions about your preferences and palliative care options are essential, so you can focus on what matters most to you.

13. **Engage Family Support**: Don't hesitate to involve your loved ones in your journey. They can provide emotional support and actively participate in your care, which can be reassuring during these challenging times.

Remember that you're not alone in facing these emotional challenges. By reaching out for professional help, connecting with others who understand your experience, and practicing self-compassion, you can effectively address anxiety and depression while navigating your brain cancer journey. Your emotional well-being is an essential component of your overall health and quality of life.

Finding Joy and Gratitude in the Present Moment

Finding joy and gratitude in the present moment is a powerful practice, especially for brain cancer patients, as it can bring comfort and improve their overall well-being. Here are some strategies tailored to the unique challenges faced by brain cancer patients:

Mindfulness Meditation

- **Start Each Day with Gratitude:** Begin your day by reflecting on the things you are grateful for. It could be the support of loved ones, a beautiful sunrise, or simply the gift of another day.

- **Keep a Gratitude Journal:** Maintain a journal where you jot down things you're grateful for each day. It could be as simple as a tasty meal, a kind word, or a moment of peace.

- **Mindful Breathing and Body Scan:** Practice mindfulness meditation with a focus on your breath. Inhale deeply, and as you exhale, imagine releasing any tension or negative thoughts. Follow this with a body scan to relax and bring awareness to different parts of your body.

- **Embrace the Five Senses:** Engage your senses mindfully. Explore the world through touch, taste, smell, sight, and sound. Even the simplest sensations can bring moments of joy and gratitude.

- **Gratitude Walks:** Take short walks and consciously observe the beauty around you. Notice the colors of the flowers, the warmth of the sun on your skin, or the sound of birds singing. Express gratitude for these sensory experiences.

- **Connect with Loved Ones:** Spend quality time with family and friends who bring joy to your life. Share your feelings of gratitude with them and let them know how much you appreciate their presence.

- **Celebrate Small Achievements:** Recognize and celebrate your daily accomplishments, no matter how minor they may seem. Each step, each meal, and each moment of joy is an achievement worth celebrating.

- **Create a Gratitude Collage:** Collect images, quotes, or words that remind you of the things you're grateful for. Create a visual collage that you can look at when you need a boost of positivity.

- **Support Groups and Community:** Join brain cancer support groups or communities where you can connect with others who understand your journey. Sharing your experiences and receiving support can foster a sense of gratitude for the bonds you form.

- **Practice Loving-Kindness Meditation:** Engage in loving-kindness meditation, directing well-wishes and compassion towards yourself, loved ones, and even those who have supported your medical journey.

- **Find Joy in Hobbies:** Dedicate time to hobbies and activities that bring you joy, whether it's painting, reading, gardening, or listening to music. Engaging in these activities can be a source of gratitude and comfort.

- **Nature Connection:** Spend time outdoors and connect with the natural world. Whether it's a park, garden, or your own backyard, nature has a way of inspiring gratitude and wonder.

- **Volunteer or Help Others:** Offering your time and support to others in need can bring immense joy and gratitude. It allows you to see the positive impact you have on the lives of others.

- **Mindful Reflection:** At the end of the day, reflect on the moments of joy and gratitude you experienced. It can be a few simple highlights that remind you of the beauty in your life.

- **Seek Professional Support:** If you find it challenging to cultivate gratitude and joy due to the emotional weight of your condition, consider working with a therapist or counselor who specializes in cancer patients' emotional well-being.

Embracing joy and gratitude in the present moment can be a profound source of comfort and positivity for brain cancer patients. It allows you to focus on the beauty and love that still exist in your life, even amid the challenges you face.

Mindfulness for Better Sleep

Mindfulness can be a valuable practice for improving sleep in brain cancer patients. Sleep disturbances are common among cancer patients, and mindfulness techniques can help promote relaxation, reduce anxiety, and enhance overall sleep quality. Here are some mindfulness strategies specifically tailored to support better sleep for brain cancer patients:

Mindful Breathing:

- **Pre-Sleep Routine**: Develop a pre-sleep mindfulness routine. Find a quiet and comfortable place where you can sit or lie down. Take a few moments to focus on your breath. Inhale slowly and deeply through your nose, then exhale through your mouth. Let go of any racing thoughts as you concentrate on your breath.

- **Body Scan:** Conduct a body scan meditation before bedtime. Pay attention to each part of your body, releasing tension and discomfort. This practice can help you relax physically and mentally.

Guided Imagery:

- **Soothing Scenes:** Use guided imagery to create a peaceful mental scene that promotes sleep. Imagine a tranquil place, such as a calm beach, a serene forest, or a cozy cabin. Visualize the details, sounds, and sensations of this peaceful place.

- **Progressive Relaxation**: Combine guided imagery with progressive muscle relaxation. Start from your toes and work your way up to your head, consciously relaxing each muscle group. As you do this, let go of any physical tension that may be interfering with your sleep.

Mindful Thoughts and Emotions:

- **Mindful Acknowledgment**: As you lie in bed, if anxious or racing thoughts intrude, acknowledge them without judgment. Simply label them as thoughts, and then gently return your focus to your breath. This practice can help you detach from worrisome thoughts.

- **Positive Affirmations**: Before sleep, remind yourself of positive affirmations. These can be personal, such as "I am at peace," "I am safe," or "I am supported." Repeating these affirmations can foster a sense of emotional security.

4. Evening Rituals:

- **Technology Detox**: Avoid exposure to screens (phones, tablets, computers) at least an hour before bedtime. The blue light emitted by screens can interfere with the production of melatonin, a hormone that regulates sleep.

- **Warm Bath**: Consider taking a warm bath before bed. The change in body temperature can promote relaxation and signal the body that it's time to wind down.

5. Mindful Tea or Snack:

- **Herbal Tea**: Enjoy a cup of caffeine-free herbal tea, such as chamomile or lavender, which can have calming properties. Practice mindfulness as you savor each sip.

- **Light Snack**: If hunger is interfering with sleep, have a light and healthy snack like a banana or a small handful of almonds. Eat mindfully, savoring each bite.

6. Yoga and Gentle Stretching:

- **Bed Yoga**: Engage in gentle yoga or stretching exercises that can be done in bed. These movements can relax your muscles and prepare your body for restful sleep.

7. Sleep Environment:

- **Comfort and Darkness**: Ensure your sleep environment is comfortable and as dark as possible. Use blackout curtains and consider an eye mask if necessary.

- **Comfortable Mattress and Bedding**: Invest in a comfortable mattress and bedding that supports a good night's sleep.

8. Sleep Schedule:

- **Consistent Routine**: Try to maintain a consistent sleep schedule. Going to bed and waking up at the same times each day helps regulate your body's internal clock.

- **Limit Naps:** While short naps can be rejuvenating, avoid long daytime naps that might interfere with nighttime sleep.

It's important to remember that improving sleep with mindfulness is a gradual process. It may take time to see significant results. Be patient with yourself and maintain a consistent mindfulness practice. Additionally, consult with your healthcare team or a sleep specialist if sleep problems persist or worsen. They can offer further guidance and interventions specific to your condition.

Coping with emotional challenges as a brain cancer patient is a vital aspect of your journey. Whether you're addressing anxiety and depression, seeking joy and gratitude, or improving your sleep with mindfulness, these strategies can help you navigate the emotional complexities of your condition. Always consult with your healthcare team for personalized guidance and support to ensure that your chosen methods align with your specific needs and treatment plan.

Chapter 10

Mindfulness in Everyday Life

Living with brain cancer can be challenging, but integrating mindfulness into your daily life can offer comfort and support, helping you navigate your journey with greater ease. This chapter explores how to apply mindfulness to your interactions with loved ones, incorporate mindfulness into daily activities, and maintain this practice beyond treatment.

Mindful Communication with Loved Ones

Practicing mindful communication with loved ones as a brain cancer patient is a powerful way to strengthen relationships, enhance emotional well-being, and promote a sense of connection during challenging times. Here are some strategies and principles for mindful communication:

1. Active Listening:

- When your loved ones are speaking, practice active listening. This means giving them your full attention without interrupting, judging, or formulating responses in your mind.

2. Non-Judgmental Presence:

- Approach conversations without judgment. Mindfulness encourages being present with an open heart and an attitude of acceptance. Allow your loved ones to express themselves freely.

3. Mindful Speaking:

- Before speaking, take a moment to pause and consider your words. Be mindful of your tone and intention. Avoid saying things impulsively that you might regret.

4. Express Gratitude:

- Share your appreciation and gratitude for your loved ones. Let them know how much their support means to you. Expressing gratitude fosters a positive and nurturing atmosphere.

5. Speak from the Heart:

- Share your feelings and thoughts honestly. Be open about your emotional experiences, fears, and hopes. Vulnerability can deepen connections.

6. Acknowledge Emotions:

- Recognize and validate your emotions and those of your loved ones. It's okay to feel a wide range of emotions, and mindfulness encourages embracing these feelings without judgment.

7. Mindful Breathing:

- During conversations, use mindful breathing techniques to stay grounded and present. If emotions become overwhelming, take a few deep breaths to regain your composure.

8. Empathetic Communication:

- Show empathy and understanding for the feelings and concerns of your loved ones. Reflect back their emotions and let them know you hear and care about their experiences.

9. Patience and Presence:

- Be patient and fully present in your interactions. If your condition affects your energy or focus, communicate this with love and gratitude for their understanding.

10. Communicate Your Needs:

- It's essential to communicate your needs clearly and honestly. Let your loved ones know how they can support you best. Mindful communication encourages you to express your needs without blame or criticism.

11. Mindful Conflict Resolution:

- If conflicts arise, approach them mindfully. Focus on the issue at hand, not past grievances. Practice active listening, express your feelings with respect, and work towards a solution together.

12. Share Mindfulness Practices:

- Invite your loved ones to join you in mindfulness practices like meditation or deep breathing exercises. This can be a way to bond and enhance your well-being together.

13. Reconnect with Memories:

- Share memories and stories from the past that hold sentimental value. Revisiting cherished moments can create a sense of connection and joy.

14. Compassionate Self-Talk:

- Practice self-compassion in your communication. Be gentle with yourself, acknowledging your courage and strength throughout your journey.

15. Set Boundaries:

- Recognize your limits and communicate your boundaries when necessary. Your loved ones will appreciate your honesty and respect for your well-being.

Mindful communication can create a supportive and empathetic environment for brain cancer patients and their loved ones. It encourages deeper connections and a sense of togetherness during the challenging journey of living with a brain cancer diagnosis.

Applying Mindfulness to Daily Activities

Applying mindfulness to daily activities can be a transformative practice for brain cancer patients. Mindfulness allows you to be fully present in each moment, fostering a sense of calm, reducing stress, and enhancing your overall well-being. Here are ways to incorporate mindfulness into your daily life:

1. Morning Routine:

- Start your day mindfully. As you wake up, take a few deep breaths and set a positive intention for the day. Be aware of the sensations as you wash your face, brush your teeth, and get dressed.

2. Mindful Eating:

- Pay full attention to your meals. Savor the flavors, textures, and aromas of the food. Chew slowly and enjoy each bite. Eating mindfully can help with digestion and enhance your connection with food.

3. Deep Breathing:

- Incorporate mindful breathing into your daily activities. Pause throughout the day to take a few deep breaths. Focus on the sensation of the breath entering and leaving your body.

4. Walking Meditation:

- If possible, practice walking meditation. Take slow, deliberate steps, paying attention to each movement. Be mindful of the sensation of your feet touching the ground.

5. Mindful Shower:

- Use your shower as an opportunity for mindfulness. Feel the warm water against your skin, notice the sensation of cleansing, and be present in the moment.

6. Mindful Driving or Commuting:

- While driving or commuting, refrain from multitasking. Pay attention to the road, your surroundings, and the act of driving. Use red lights or traffic jams as reminders to take mindful breaths.

7. Mindful Technology Use:

- Be conscious of how you use technology. Instead of mindlessly scrolling through your phone or computer, take breaks to engage in mindful breathing and body scans.

8. Mindful Cleaning:

- Transform household chores into opportunities for mindfulness. As you clean, feel the sensations of your body moving, the texture of surfaces, and the sound of cleaning.

9. Mindful Resting:

- When resting or lying down, practice a body scan. Pay attention to each part of your body, relaxing any areas of tension.

10. Mindful Appreciation:

- Throughout the day, take moments to appreciate the small joys in life. It could be the warmth of the sun on your skin, the laughter of loved ones, or the beauty of nature.

11. Mindful Journaling:

- Keep a mindfulness journal. Reflect on your experiences, emotions, and moments of gratitude. Journaling can help you process your journey and maintain a mindful perspective.

12. Mindful Moments of Solitude:

- Create moments of solitude to meditate or simply sit quietly. These moments allow you to reconnect with your inner self and find inner peace.

13. Engage the Senses:

- Engage your senses mindfully. Whether it's the taste of your favorite tea, the texture of a cozy blanket, or the sound of soothing music, appreciate the sensory experiences in your life.

14. Bedtime Routine:

- End your day with a mindfulness practice. Reflect on the positive aspects of the day, let go of any worries, and prepare your mind for restful sleep.

15. Self-Compassion:

- Throughout the day, practice self-compassion. Be kind and gentle with yourself. Acknowledge your strength, resilience, and the courage it takes to face your journey.

Incorporating mindfulness into your daily activities can help you find peace, reduce stress, and improve your overall quality of life as a brain cancer patient. Mindfulness allows you to embrace each moment with gratitude and awareness.

Integrating mindfulness into your daily life as a brain cancer patient can enhance your well-being and help you navigate the challenges of your journey. Whether you're communicating with loved ones, applying mindfulness to daily activities, or maintaining your practice beyond treatment, mindfulness can be a valuable resource. Always consult with your healthcare team for personalized guidance to ensure that your mindfulness practice aligns with your specific needs and treatment plan.

Chapter 11

Building a Supportive Community

Cancer can be a challenging journey, and building a supportive community can provide emotional strength and encouragement. This guide will explore how to connect with supportive communities, including joining support groups, connecting with other brain cancer patients, and recognizing the vital role caregivers play in your mindfulness journey.

Joining Support Groups

Support groups offer a safe and welcoming space for cancer patients to share their experiences, seek advice, and gain emotional support. Consider these steps when joining a support group:

- **Find Local or Online Groups**: Look for local cancer support groups in your area or explore online communities where you can connect with individuals who understand your experiences.

- **Attend Meetings Regularly**: Commit to attending meetings regularly, whether in person or virtually. Consistent participation can help you build stronger connections within the group.

- **Share Your Story**: Be open to sharing your own experiences and listening to the stories of others. This mutual exchange can create a sense of community and understanding.

- **Seek Professional Guidance:** Some support groups are facilitated by mental health professionals who can provide valuable guidance and resources. This can be particularly helpful in navigating emotional challenges.

Here are some reasons why you might consider joining a support group:

1. Emotional Support:

- Support groups offer a safe and understanding environment where you can express your feelings, fears, and concerns without judgment. This emotional support can be invaluable during your brain cancer journey.

2. Shared Experiences:

- In a support group, you'll meet others who are going through or have gone through similar experiences. Sharing your stories and hearing theirs can help you feel less alone and more understood.

3. Practical Advice:

- Support groups often provide practical advice and tips for managing the challenges of brain cancer, from treatment side effects to coping with emotions.

4. Coping Strategies:

- Members of support groups share coping strategies they've found helpful, including mindfulness techniques, stress management, and methods for dealing with anxiety or depression.

5. Information and Resources:

- Support groups can provide access to valuable information about treatment options, clinical trials, and resources for brain cancer patients.

6. Building Friendships:

- Many people form lasting friendships in support groups. These connections can provide companionship and a sense of community during your journey.

7. Reducing Isolation:

- Brain cancer can be an isolating experience, but joining a support group helps counter that isolation. You'll be surrounded by people who understand your journey and can offer comfort.

8. Sense of Empowerment:

- By participating in a support group, you can regain a sense of control and empowerment in your life. You'll learn how to advocate for yourself and make informed decisions about your care.

9. Reduced Stress:

- Sharing your concerns and hearing from others can reduce the stress and anxiety often associated with brain cancer. It can be a relief to know you're not alone in your feelings.

10. Caregiver Support:

- Support groups aren't just for patients. Many offer separate sessions or groups for caregivers and loved ones. This helps them cope with their unique challenges and find support too.

11. Avenues for Expression:

- Support groups provide a platform to express your feelings and concerns. Whether it's through speaking, writing, or creative activities, it can be cathartic to share.

12. Hope and Positivity:

- Being part of a support group allows you to witness others' journeys and see positive outcomes, which can inspire hope and a sense of optimism.

13. Healthcare Team Referrals:

- Many healthcare providers can refer you to local support groups. They may have insights into which groups are the best fit for your needs.

14. Online Support:

- If attending in-person meetings is difficult due to health constraints, consider online support groups. These virtual communities offer many of the same benefits and can be a convenient option.

Remember that you're not alone on this journey. Joining a support group can provide you with a network of understanding individuals who can help you navigate the challenges of brain cancer and offer you a sense of community and support.

Connecting with Other Brain Cancer Patients

Connecting with other brain cancer patients can be a source of tremendous support and understanding during your journey. Here are some ways to connect with fellow patients:

1. Support Groups:

- Look for local or online support groups specifically for brain cancer patients. These groups provide a space for sharing experiences, challenges, and coping strategies.

2. Online Communities:

- Join online forums, social media groups, or platforms dedicated to brain cancer. These communities allow you to connect with patients worldwide, share stories, and offer and receive support.

3. Local Events:

- Attend local events, workshops, or seminars related to brain cancer. These gatherings can provide opportunities to meet other patients and their families face to face.

4. Patient Advocacy Groups:

- Explore patient advocacy organizations or charities focused on brain cancer. They often have resources for connecting with other patients and participating in events or programs.

5. Hospital or Clinic Programs:

- Inquire at your treatment center about any patient programs or support initiatives they may offer. Many hospitals have support groups or events for cancer patients.

6. Online Blogs and Personal Stories:

- Read and engage with online blogs and personal stories of brain cancer patients. Many individuals share their journeys, insights, and tips, offering a sense of connection.

7. Social Media:

- Utilize social media platforms to connect with fellow patients. Search for relevant hashtags and join discussions on platforms like Twitter, Instagram, or Facebook.

8. Local Cancer Organizations:

- Reach out to local cancer organizations, as they may have information about support groups, events, or peer-to-peer support for brain cancer patients.

9. Hospital Resources:

- Consult with your healthcare team to inquire about any patient support resources or contacts they can provide.

10. Attend Brain Cancer Awareness Events:

- Participate in brain cancer awareness events and walks. These gatherings often bring together patients, caregivers, and advocates.

11. Reach Out to Supportive Care Services:

- Hospitals and treatment centers typically have supportive care services that can connect you with patient groups or individuals facing similar challenges.

12. Connect with Caregivers:

- Engage with caregivers and loved ones of brain cancer patients. Their experiences and insights can offer a unique perspective and understanding.

13. Attend Conferences:

- Attend cancer conferences or events where brain cancer is a topic of discussion. These gatherings can provide opportunities to network and connect.

14. Volunteer:

- Consider volunteering for brain cancer-related organizations or events. It's a way to give back and connect with other patients and advocates.

15. Personal Connections:

- Share your journey and experiences with friends, family, and coworkers. They may know someone who can connect you with other brain cancer patients.

Connecting with other brain cancer patients can be a source of comfort, inspiration, and valuable information. It's an opportunity to share your experiences, learn from others, and find a sense of community on this challenging journey.

The Role of Caregivers in the Mindfulness Journey

Caregivers play a vital role in the mindfulness journey of a brain cancer patient. Mindfulness not only benefits the patient but also extends to the caregivers, helping them cope with the challenges of providing care and support. Here's how caregivers can contribute to and benefit from the mindfulness journey:

1. Emotional Support:

- Caregivers can provide emotional support by encouraging mindfulness practices and participating in them alongside the patient. Being a source of understanding and empathy can create a nurturing environment for mindfulness.

2. Encouragement:

- Caregivers can motivate the patient to maintain their mindfulness routine, whether it's meditation, deep breathing, or other practices. Gentle reminders and encouragement can be very helpful.

3. Active Listening:

- Mindful listening is a key component of caregiving. Caregivers can actively listen to the patient's thoughts and feelings without judgment, offering a compassionate presence.

4. Mindful Presence:

- Caregivers can practice mindfulness themselves to remain fully present during their caregiving tasks. This can reduce stress and enhance the quality of care they provide.

5. Joining Mindfulness Practices:

- Caregivers can participate in mindfulness practices with the patient. This not only provides companionship but also helps caregivers manage their own stress and emotions.

6. Respite for Self-Care:

- Caregivers need to take breaks and practice self-care. Mindfulness can help them recharge and reduce the burnout associated with caregiving.

7. Stress Management:

- Caregivers can use mindfulness techniques to manage their stress and anxiety. This benefits both the caregiver and the patient, as a calm and composed caregiver is more effective.

8. Understanding Boundaries:

- Mindfulness can help caregivers set and maintain healthy boundaries. Understanding their limitations and ensuring self-care is crucial for long-term caregiving.

9. Compassion and Self-Compassion:

- Caregivers can cultivate compassion, both for the patient and for themselves. Self-compassion is especially important for caregivers to avoid burnout.

10. Communication:

- Caregivers can practice mindful communication. This includes empathetic listening, clear and compassionate expression, and non-judgmental conversations with the patient.

11. Coping with Grief:

- Grief and loss are common in the caregiving journey. Mindfulness can help caregivers navigate the emotions associated with loss in a healthy and constructive way.

12. Advocacy:

- Caregivers can advocate for the patient's well-being and encourage them to express their needs, concerns, and preferences to the healthcare team.

13. Learning Together:

- Caregivers can learn about mindfulness alongside the patient. This shared journey can enhance the caregiving relationship and provide both parties with a common tool for managing the challenges.

14. Seeking Support:

- Caregivers can seek support for themselves through caregiver support groups, therapy, or counseling. Connecting with other caregivers can offer valuable insights and emotional support.

15. Encouraging Independence:

- Caregivers can use mindfulness to support the patient's independence where possible. Encouraging self-care and self-management can boost the patient's confidence and well-being.

The role of caregivers in the mindfulness journey of a brain cancer patient is multifaceted. They offer not only physical care but also emotional support, understanding, and a shared commitment to well-being. Mindfulness benefits not just the patient but also the caregivers, fostering resilience, reducing stress, and enhancing the quality of care provided.

Building a supportive community as a cancer patient is essential for emotional well-being and resilience. By joining support groups, connecting with fellow brain cancer patients, and involving caregivers in your mindfulness journey, you can create a network of understanding and strength to navigate the challenges that cancer presents. Always consult with your healthcare team and support networks for personalized guidance to ensure that your chosen methods align with your specific needs and treatment plan.

Chapter 12

The Power of Resilience

Facing cancer, particularly brain cancer, can be an incredibly daunting journey. In this guide, we'll explore the concept of resilience, drawing inspiration from stories of brain cancer survivors who have triumphed over adversity. We'll also delve into finding inner peace amidst the storm and moving forward with mindfulness as you navigate your own path to recovery and well-being.

Stories of Brain Cancer Survivors

Stories of brain cancer survivors are often inspiring and provide hope for those facing similar challenges. While I don't have access to specific real-life stories of brain cancer survivors, I can provide you with a general overview of what some survivors have experienced. Keep in mind that each person's journey with cancer is unique, and the outcomes can vary.

1. **Valerie Harper**: The famous actress Valerie Harper was diagnosed with terminal brain cancer in 2013 and given just a few months to live. However, she defied the odds and continued to live for several more years, becoming an advocate for cancer research and raising

awareness about the disease. She demonstrated incredible resilience and a positive outlook throughout her battle.

2. **John McCain:** The late Senator John McCain was diagnosed with glioblastoma, one of the most aggressive forms of brain cancer, in 2017. Despite his diagnosis, he continued to serve in the Senate and remained active in public life while undergoing treatment. His strength and determination were an inspiration to many.

3. **Maria Menounos:** Television personality Maria Menounos was diagnosed with a benign brain tumor in 2017. She underwent surgery to remove the tumor and has since been open about her

journey and the importance of early detection and seeking medical help.

4. **David Bailey**: David Bailey, a motivational speaker and musician, was diagnosed with an aggressive form of brain cancer in 2007. He not only survived but also continued to pursue his passion for music and inspire others through his story of resilience.

5. **Liz Salmi**: Liz Salmi is a brain cancer survivor who became an advocate for patients and caregivers. She shares her journey and offers support and resources to those dealing with brain cancer through her blog and work with organizations like the National Brain Tumor Society.

6. **Senator Ted Kennedy**: The late Senator Ted Kennedy was diagnosed with a malignant glioma, a type of brain tumor, in 2008. Despite his diagnosis, he continued to work on legislation and healthcare reform, serving as an advocate for cancer research and awareness.

7. **Paula Franzese**: Paula Franzese, a law professor, and real estate developer, was diagnosed with a brain tumor in 2017. She underwent surgery and treatment, and her resilience in the face of adversity serves as an inspiration to many. She has also been actively involved in fundraising for brain cancer research.

8. **Matt Newman**: Matt Newman, a former Marine and avid athlete, was diagnosed with an aggressive form of brain cancer in 2013. He has since become an advocate for cancer research and has completed various endurance challenges to raise awareness and funds for brain cancer research.

9. **Mark Ruffalo**: The well-known actor Mark Ruffalo had a benign brain tumor removed in 2001. He has been open about his experience and used his platform to raise awareness about brain tumors and the importance of regular check-ups.

10. **Lauren Hill**: Lauren Hill was a young basketball player who was diagnosed with a rare and aggressive form of brain cancer called DIPG. Despite her diagnosis, she fulfilled her dream of playing in a college basketball game and raised awareness for pediatric brain cancer. She passed away in 2015, but her legacy continues through the Lauren Hill Award, which supports pediatric cancer research.

11. **John S. McCain III**: In addition to Senator John McCain, his father, Admiral John S. McCain Jr., was also a brain cancer survivor. He was diagnosed with a glioblastoma multiforme in the late 1970s and underwent surgery and treatment, ultimately living for several more years.

These stories highlight the strength, resilience, and determination of brain cancer survivors. Their experiences also emphasize the importance of early detection, advanced medical treatments, and the critical role of support from family, friends, and the broader community in the journey to recovery.

It's important to remember that every brain cancer survivor's story is unique, and their experiences can serve as a source of hope and inspiration for others facing this challenging diagnosis.

Finding Inner Peace Amidst the Storm

Finding inner peace amidst the storm of a serious illness like brain cancer can be an incredibly challenging journey, but it's also a path that can bring a sense of tranquility and resilience in the face of adversity. Here are some steps and strategies that may help:

1. **Accept Your Emotions:** It's entirely normal to experience a wide range of emotions when dealing with a serious illness. Allow yourself to feel what you're feeling without judgment. Give yourself permission to grieve, be angry, or be scared. Acknowledging your emotions is an important first step.

2. **Mindfulness and Meditation:** These practices can help you stay present in the moment and reduce anxiety. Mindfulness can teach you to observe your thoughts and feelings without becoming overwhelmed by them. Consider attending mindfulness-based stress reduction (MBSR) programs or using meditation apps that are designed for managing stress.

3. **Stay Informed but Not Obsessed:** Knowledge can be empowering, but it's important not to become consumed by the details of your illness. Stay informed about your condition, treatments, and options, but avoid excessive Googling or dwelling on worst-case scenarios.

4. **Support System**: Surround yourself with people who love and care for you. Sharing your feelings with close friends and family can provide comfort and emotional support. Consider joining support groups specifically for cancer patients or those facing similar challenges. Connecting with others who understand your journey can be tremendously comforting.

5. **Set Realistic Goals**: Set small, achievable goals for yourself. These goals can provide a sense of purpose and accomplishment. Whether it's completing a puzzle, taking a short walk, or reading a book, these small wins can bring a sense of satisfaction.

6. **Healthy Lifestyle Choices**: To the extent possible, maintain a healthy lifestyle. Eating a balanced diet, staying physically active (within the limits set by your healthcare provider), and getting adequate sleep can all contribute to your overall well-being.

7. **Spirituality or Faith**: If you have religious or spiritual beliefs, these can provide a sense of solace and purpose. Many people find comfort in their faith during challenging times. Seek spiritual guidance or connect with your religious community if it aligns with your beliefs.

8. **Seek Professional Help**: Consider seeing a mental health professional, such as a therapist or counselor, who specializes in

working with individuals dealing with chronic illness. They can provide valuable coping strategies and emotional support.

9. **Creative Outlets**: Engaging in creative activities like art, writing, or music can be therapeutic. Expressing yourself through creativity can be a way to release emotions and find solace.

10. **Gratitude**: Cultivate a sense of gratitude for the things that bring joy and meaning to your life. Regularly reflecting on the things you are thankful for can shift your focus away from the challenges you face.

Remember, finding inner peace is a unique and ongoing journey for each individual. It's okay to have difficult moments, and it's okay to ask for help when needed. The process may involve several steps forward and sometimes a step or two backward. But over time, with persistence and the right support, many people do find a sense of peace amidst life's storms.

Resilience is not about the absence of difficulties; it's about your ability to navigate and grow through them. The power of resilience, drawn from the stories of survivors, the pursuit of inner peace, and the incorporation of mindfulness, can provide you with the strength and determination to face your brain cancer diagnosis and emerge stronger on the other side. Always consult with your healthcare team and support networks for personalized guidance to ensure that your

chosen methods align with your specific

needs and treatment plan.

Conclusion

As we draw the final pages of "Mindfulness Meditation for Brain Cancer Patients: Finding Inner Peace Amidst the Storm" to a close, we are reminded that this journey is not one that ends with the turning of a last page. Rather, it is a lifelong odyssey, a commitment to the continuous practice of mindfulness and a pursuit of inner peace.

Through the pages of this book, we have explored the power of mindfulness as a source of strength and resilience for brain cancer patients. We have shared the stories of individuals who have courageously embraced this practice, finding solace and renewed purpose in the face of immense challenges.

In the realm of brain cancer, where the storms may be fierce and the path uncertain, we have witnessed the incredible potential of the human spirit to find calm amidst chaos, to discover hope amidst despair, and to experience healing amidst pain.

As you take the lessons learned from this book into your own life, remember that mindfulness is a journey of a lifetime. It is a practice that can provide comfort, clarity, and resilience. Embrace each moment with awareness and compassion. Allow your journey to be a testament to the strength and grace within you.

May this book serve as a beacon of hope, a guide in times of darkness, and a reminder that, even amidst the most turbulent storms, inner peace is an achievable destination. As you continue your voyage, know that you are not alone. Together, we walk the path of mindfulness, finding inner peace amidst the storm, and nurturing the light of resilience and serenity within our hearts.

www.ingramcontent.com/pod-product-compliance
Lightning Source LLC
Chambersburg PA
CBHW050805260726
48660CB00004B/1253